RENAL DISEASE DIET COOKBOOK FOR WOMEN

20 DELICIOUS LOW SODIUM, POTASSIUM, PHOSPHORUS RENAL DIET FOR WOMEN

LAURA PHOEBE

COPYRIGHT

TABLE OF CONTENT

INTRODUCTION

In a cozy kitchen nestled between fragrant herb pots, Lily discovered the magic of flavors that danced without missing a beat. With apron strings tied and pots simmering, Lily, a spirited chef, embarked on a culinary journey to create a symphony of nourishment for her dear friend, Emma. Emma, battling kidney disease, found solace in Lily's delicious concoctions.

The kitchen became a canvas where Lily blended colors of health with fresh produce and low-potassium wonders. Together, they crafted a cookbook, not just filled with recipes, but a tale of resilience and friendship. Each page unfolded a chapter of savory delights, transforming Emma's dietary restrictions into a celebration of taste and vitality. The aroma of ginger and rosemary wafted through the air, symbolizing a journey that embraced life's challenges with a pinch of spice and a dash of love. Emma's kitchen not only fostered well-being but became a haven where every recipe whispered a story of triumph over adversity.

DELICIOUS RENAL DIET COOKBOOK FOR WOMEN

Grilled Lemon Herb Chicken

Prep Time: 20 minutes

Ingredients:

- 4 boneless, skinless chicken breasts
- 2 tablespoons olive oil
- 2 tablespoons fresh lemon juice
- 2 cloves garlic, minced
- 1 teaspoon dried oregano
- 1 teaspoon dried thyme
- Salt and pepper to taste
- Lemon wedges for garnish

Prep Steps:

Marinate Chicken:

In a bowl, mix olive oil, lemon juice, minced garlic, dried oregano, dried thyme, salt, and pepper to create the marinade.

Prepare Chicken:

Place the chicken breasts in a resealable plastic bag or shallow dish. Pour the marinade over the chicken, ensuring each piece is well-coated. Seal the bag or cover the dish and refrigerate for at least 15 minutes.

Preheat Grill:

Preheat your grill to medium-high heat.

Grill Chicken:

Remove the chicken from the marinade and place it on the preheated grill. Grill each side for 6-8 minutes or until the internal temperature reaches 165°F (74°C) and there are nice grill marks.

Rest and Garnish:

Allow the grilled chicken to rest for a few minutes before serving. Garnish with lemon wedges.

Nutritional Value (per serving):

- Calories: 250 kcal
- Protein: 30g
- Fat: 12g
- Carbohydrates: 2g
- Fiber: 1g
- Sodium: 80mg
- Potassium: 300mg
- Phosphorus: 200mg

Note:

This kidney-friendly grilled lemon herb chicken is a delicious and low-phosphorus option for those with renal concerns. The lemon adds a refreshing zing, while the herbs provide savory depth. Adjust salt according to your dietary needs, and pair it with a side of steamed vegetables or a kidney-friendly salad for a well-balanced meal. Always consult with a healthcare professional or dietitian to ensure the recipe aligns with your specific dietary requirements.

Quinoa Salad with Cucumber and Mint

Prep Time: 15 minutes

Ingredients:

- 1 cup quinoa, rinsed
- 2 cups water
- 1 cucumber, diced
- 1/4 cup fresh mint leaves, chopped
- 1/4 cup red onion, finely diced

- 2 tablespoons olive oil
- 2 tablespoons fresh lemon juice
- Salt and pepper to taste

Prep Steps:

Cook Quinoa:

In a medium saucepan, combine quinoa and water. Bring to a boil, then reduce heat to low, cover, and simmer for 12-15 minutes, or until quinoa is cooked and water is absorbed. Let it cool.

Prepare Vegetables:

In a large bowl, combine diced cucumber, chopped mint, and finely diced red onion.

Combine Quinoa and Vegetables:

Add the cooled quinoa to the bowl with the vegetables.

Make Dressing:

In a small bowl, whisk together olive oil, fresh lemon juice, salt, and pepper to create the dressing.

Toss and Chill:

Pour the dressing over the quinoa mixture and toss gently to coat evenly. Refrigerate for at least 30 minutes to let the flavors meld.

Nutritional Value (per serving):

- Calories: 220 kcal
- Protein: 6g
- Fat: 8g
- Carbohydrates: 32g
- Fiber: 4g
- Sodium: 10mg
- Potassium: 180mg
- Phosphorus: 120mg

Note:

This refreshing quinoa salad with cucumber and mint is a kidney-friendly delight. Quinoa provides a protein boost, while the cucumber adds a crisp texture and the mint imparts a burst of freshness. The olive oil and lemon dressing enhances the flavors without compromising renal health. Adjust salt and portion sizes based on your dietary needs, and feel free to customize with additional kidney-friendly vegetables. Always consult with a healthcare professional or dietitian for personalized dietary advice.

Baked Salmon with Dill

Prep Time: 25 minutes

Ingredients:

- 4 salmon fillets
- 2 tablespoons olive oil
- 2 tablespoons fresh lemon juice
- 2 cloves garlic, minced
- 2 tablespoons fresh dill, chopped
- Salt and pepper to taste
- Lemon slices for garnish

Prep Steps:

Preheat Oven:

Preheat your oven to 375°F (190°C).

Prepare Salmon:

Pat the salmon fillets dry with a paper towel and place them on a baking sheet lined with parchment paper.

Make Marinade:

In a small bowl, mix together olive oil, fresh lemon juice, minced garlic, chopped dill, salt, and pepper to create the marinade.

Marinate Salmon:

Brush the salmon fillets with the marinade, ensuring they are well-coated. Allow them to marinate for at least 10 minutes.

Bake Salmon:

Bake the salmon in the preheated oven for 15-18 minutes or until the fish flakes easily with a fork.

Garnish and Serve:

Remove the salmon from the oven, garnish with lemon slices and additional dill if desired, and serve.

Nutritional Value (per serving):

- Calories: 300 kcal
- Protein: 30g
- Fat: 18g
- Carbohydrates: 1g
- Fiber: 0g
- Sodium: 70mg
- Potassium: 450mg
- Phosphorus: 250mg

Note:

This baked salmon with dill is a kidney-friendly dish rich in omega-3 fatty acids. The dill adds a delightful herbaceous flavor, complementing the natural taste of the salmon. Adjust salt according to your dietary needs. Serve this dish with a side of steamed vegetables or a low-potassium salad for a balanced meal. As with any dietary changes, consult with a healthcare professional or dietitian to ensure it aligns with your specific renal requirements.

Vegetable Stir-Fry

Prep Time: 20 minutes

Ingredients:

- 2 cups broccoli florets
- 1 bell pepper, thinly sliced
- 1 carrot, julienned

- 1 cup snap peas, trimmed
- 2 tablespoons low-sodium soy sauce
- 1 tablespoon sesame oil
- 1 tablespoon olive oil
- 2 cloves garlic, minced
- 1 teaspoon fresh ginger, grated
- 1 tablespoon rice vinegar
- 1 tablespoon low-sodium vegetable broth
- Sesame seeds for garnish (optional)
- Brown rice or quinoa for serving

Prep Steps:

Prepare Vegetables:

Wash and chop broccoli, bell pepper, carrot, and snap peas.

Heat Oils:

In a large wok or skillet, heat olive oil and sesame oil over medium-high heat.

Sauté Aromatics:

Add minced garlic and grated ginger to the hot oil. Sauté for 1-2 minutes until fragrant.

Stir-Fry Vegetables:

Add broccoli, bell pepper, carrot, and snap peas to the wok. Stir-fry for 5-7 minutes until vegetables are tender-crisp.

Prepare Sauce:

In a small bowl, mix low-sodium soy sauce, rice vinegar, and low-sodium vegetable broth.

Combine Sauce:

Pour the sauce over the stir-fried vegetables. Toss to coat evenly.

Garnish and Serve:

Sprinkle sesame seeds over the stir-fry if desired. Serve over brown rice or quinoa.

Nutritional Value (per serving, excluding rice/quinoa):

- Calories: 120 kcal
- Protein: 4g
- Fat: 7g
- Carbohydrates: 12g
- Fiber: 4g
- Sodium: 250mg
- Potassium: 280mg
- Phosphorus: 70mg

Note:

This vegetable stir-fry is a kidney-friendly dish that's both nutritious and delicious. Packed with colorful veggies, it provides essential nutrients with lower sodium content. Customize the vegetables based on your preferences and renal diet guidelines. Serve it over brown rice or quinoa for a complete meal. As always, consult with a healthcare professional or dietitian to ensure it aligns with your specific renal dietary requirements.

Roasted Sweet Potato Wedges

Prep Time: 30 minutes

Ingredients:

- 2 large sweet potatoes, scrubbed and cut into wedges
- 2 tablespoons olive oil
- 1 teaspoon smoked paprika
- 1/2 teaspoon garlic powder
- 1/2 teaspoon onion powder
- 1/2 teaspoon dried thyme
- Salt and pepper to taste
- Fresh parsley for garnish (optional)

Prep Steps:

Preheat Oven:

Preheat your oven to 425°F (220°C).

Prepare Sweet Potatoes:

Scrub the sweet potatoes well, leaving the skin on, and cut them into wedges of equal size.

Season Sweet Potatoes:

In a large bowl, toss sweet potato wedges with olive oil, smoked paprika, garlic powder, onion powder, dried thyme, salt, and pepper. Ensure even coating.

Arrange on Baking Sheet:

Spread the seasoned sweet potato wedges in a single layer on a baking sheet lined with parchment paper.

Roast:

Roast in the preheated oven for 25-30 minutes, flipping halfway through, or until the wedges are golden and tender.

Garnish and Serve:

Garnish with fresh parsley if desired. Serve hot.

Nutritional Value (per serving):

- Calories: 180 kcal
- Protein: 2g
- Fat: 7g
- Carbohydrates: 30g
- Fiber: 5g
- Sodium: 80mg
- Potassium: 400mg
- Phosphorus: 60mg

Note:

These roasted sweet potato wedges are a kidney-friendly alternative to traditional fries. Rich in fiber and potassium, sweet potatoes are a nutritious choice. Adjust seasonings according to your taste preferences and renal diet guidelines. Enjoy these wedges as a side dish or snack.

Consult with a healthcare professional or dietitian to ensure they fit well into your renal diet plan.

Turkey and Vegetable Skewers

Prep Time: 30 minutes

Ingredients:

- 1 pound lean turkey breast, cut into cubes
- 1 zucchini, sliced into rounds
- 1 bell pepper, cut into chunks
- 1 red onion, cut into wedges
- 2 tablespoons olive oil
- 1 tablespoon balsamic vinegar
- 1 teaspoon dried oregano
- 1 teaspoon garlic powder
- Salt and pepper to taste
- Wooden or metal skewers

Prep Steps:

Marinate Turkey:

In a bowl, combine turkey cubes with olive oil, balsamic vinegar, dried oregano, garlic powder, salt, and pepper. Allow it to marinate for at least 15 minutes.

Prepare Vegetables:

Thread marinated turkey, zucchini rounds, bell pepper chunks, and red onion wedges onto skewers, alternating for variety.

Preheat Grill:

Preheat your grill or grill pan to medium-high heat.

Grill Skewers:

Grill the skewers for 10-12 minutes, turning occasionally, or until the turkey is cooked through and vegetables are charred and tender.

Serve Hot:

Remove skewers from the grill and let them rest for a few minutes. Serve hot.

Nutritional Value (per serving):

- Calories: 220 kcal
- Protein: 25g
- Fat: 8g
- Carbohydrates: 10g
- Fiber: 2g
- Sodium: 80mg
- Potassium: 350mg
- Phosphorus: 200mg

Note:

These turkey and vegetable skewers are a kidney-friendly delight, providing lean protein and a variety of colorful veggies. The balsamic-marinated turkey adds depth of flavor without compromising renal health. Adjust seasoning according to your dietary needs. Serve with a side of low-potassium grains or a green salad for a balanced meal. As with any dietary changes, consult with a healthcare professional or dietitian to ensure it aligns with your specific renal requirements.

Mango Salsa Chicken

Prep Time: 25 minutes

Ingredients:

- 4 boneless, skinless chicken breasts
- 1 ripe mango, peeled and diced
- 1/2 red onion, finely chopped
- 1 red bell pepper, diced
- 1 jalapeño, seeded and finely chopped
- 1/4 cup fresh cilantro, chopped
- 2 tablespoons lime juice
- 1 tablespoon olive oil
- 1 teaspoon ground cumin
- Salt and pepper to taste

Prep Steps:

Prepare Chicken:

Season chicken breasts with olive oil, ground cumin, salt, and pepper. Grill or bake until fully cooked, approximately 15-18 minutes.

Make Mango Salsa:

In a bowl, combine diced mango, red onion, red bell pepper, jalapeño, cilantro, and lime juice. Mix well to create the salsa.

Serve:

Spoon the mango salsa over the cooked chicken breasts.

Nutritional Value (per serving):

- Calories: 280 kcal
- Protein: 30g
- Fat: 8g
- Carbohydrates: 25g
- Fiber: 4g
- Sodium: 70mg
- Potassium: 480mg
- Phosphorus: 250mg

Note:

This Mango Salsa Chicken is a kidney-friendly dish bursting with vibrant flavors. Mango adds a sweet twist, complementing the grilled chicken. Adjust the spiciness by modifying the amount of jalapeño. Serve this dish with a side of low-phosphorus grains or steamed vegetables for a balanced meal. Always consult with a healthcare professional or dietitian to ensure it aligns with your specific renal dietary requirements.

Spinach and Feta Stuffed Bell Peppers

Prep Time: 40 minutes

Ingredients:

- 4 large bell peppers, halved and seeds removed
- 2 cups fresh spinach, chopped
- 1 cup crumbled feta cheese
- 1 cup cooked quinoa
- 1/2 cup red onion, finely diced
- 2 cloves garlic, minced
- 1 tablespoon olive oil
- 1 teaspoon dried oregano
- Salt and pepper to taste
- 1/4 cup fresh parsley, chopped (for garnish)

Prep Steps:

Preheat Oven:

Preheat your oven to 375°F (190°C).

Prepare Bell Peppers:

Halve the bell peppers and remove the seeds. Parboil them in boiling water for 5 minutes, then drain and set aside.

Sauté Vegetables:

In a skillet, heat olive oil over medium heat. Sauté red onion and garlic until softened. Add chopped spinach and cook until wilted.

Mix Filling:

In a bowl, combine the sautéed vegetables with crumbled feta, cooked quinoa, dried oregano, salt, and pepper.

Stuff Bell Peppers:

Spoon the spinach and feta mixture into the parboiled bell peppers, pressing down gently.

Bake:

Place the stuffed bell peppers in a baking dish. Bake for 20-25 minutes or until the peppers are tender.

Garnish and Serve:

Remove from the oven, garnish with fresh parsley, and serve hot.

Nutritional Value (per serving):

- Calories: 220 kcal
- Protein: 10g
- Fat: 12g
- Carbohydrates: 20g
- Fiber: 5g
- Sodium: 350mg
- Potassium: 400mg

- Phosphorus: 150mg

Note:

These Spinach and Feta Stuffed Bell Peppers are kidney-friendly and packed with nutrients. The combination of spinach, feta, and quinoa provides a protein boost. Adjust the seasonings according to your taste preferences. Serve as a main dish or a hearty side. Always consult with a healthcare professional or dietitian to ensure it aligns with your specific renal dietary requirements.

Cauliflower Mash

Prep Time: 20 minutes

Ingredients:

- 1 large head of cauliflower, chopped into florets
- 2 cloves garlic, minced
- 2 tablespoons unsalted butter or olive oil
- 1/4 cup low-fat sour cream
- Salt and pepper to taste
- Chopped chives or parsley for garnish (optional)

Prep Steps:

Steam Cauliflower:

Place cauliflower florets in a steamer basket over boiling water. Steam for 10-12 minutes or until cauliflower is fork-tender.

Drain and Dry:

Drain the steamed cauliflower well. Pat it dry with a paper towel to remove excess moisture.

Mash Cauliflower:

In a food processor or using a hand masher, blend the cauliflower until smooth.

Sauté Garlic:

In a small pan, sauté minced garlic in butter or olive oil over medium heat until fragrant. Be careful not to brown the garlic.

Combine and Season:

Add the sautéed garlic, low-fat sour cream, salt, and pepper to the mashed cauliflower. Blend until well combined and creamy.

Adjust Consistency:

If the cauliflower mash is too thick, add a bit more sour cream or a splash of low-fat milk until you achieve your desired consistency.

Garnish and Serve:

Garnish with chopped chives or parsley if desired. Serve hot.

Nutritional Value (per serving):

- Calories: 80 kcal
- Protein: 3g

- Fat: 5g

- Carbohydrates: 8g

- Fiber: 4g

- Sodium: 70mg

- Potassium: 430mg

- Phosphorus: 70mg

Note:

Cauliflower mash is a fantastic kidney-friendly alternative to traditional mashed potatoes. It's low in potassium and phosphorus, making it suitable for renal diets. Adjust the seasoning and consistency to match your taste preferences. Serve it alongside your favorite protein for a comforting and nutritious side dish. Always consult with a healthcare professional or dietitian to ensure it aligns with your specific renal dietary requirements.

Lemon Garlic Shrimp Skewers

Prep Time: 25 minutes

Ingredients:

- 1 pound large shrimp, peeled and deveined

- 2 tablespoons olive oil

- 3 cloves garlic, minced

- Zest of 1 lemon

- 2 tablespoons fresh lemon juice

- 1 teaspoon dried oregano

- Salt and pepper to taste

- Wooden or metal skewers

Prep Steps:

Prepare Shrimp:

Rinse and pat dry the shrimp. If using wooden skewers, soak them in water for at least 15 minutes to prevent burning.

Make Marinade:

In a bowl, mix together olive oil, minced garlic, lemon zest, lemon juice, dried oregano, salt, and pepper to create the marinade.

Marinate Shrimp:

Toss the shrimp in the marinade, ensuring each piece is coated. Let it marinate for at least 10 minutes.

Skewer Shrimp:

Thread the marinated shrimp onto skewers, distributing them evenly.

Preheat Grill:

Preheat your grill or grill pan to medium-high heat.

Grill Shrimp:

Grill the shrimp skewers for 2-3 minutes per side or until the shrimp turn opaque and slightly charred.

Serve Hot:

Remove the skewers from the grill and serve immediately.

Nutritional Value (per serving):

- Calories: 180 kcal

- Protein: 24g

- Fat: 9g

- Carbohydrates: 2g

- Fiber: 0g

- Sodium: 240mg

- Potassium: 200mg

- Phosphorus: 180mg

Note:

Lemon Garlic Shrimp Skewers are a kidney-friendly delight, providing a burst of flavor without compromising renal health. The lemon and garlic add zest, while the shrimp offers a lean source of protein. Adjust salt according to your dietary needs. Serve these skewers over a bed of steamed vegetables or with a side of low-phosphorus grains for a well-balanced meal. As with any dietary changes, consult with a healthcare professional or dietitian to ensure it aligns with your specific renal requirements.

Herbed Brown Rice Pilaf

Prep Time: 35 minutes

Ingredients:

- 1 cup brown rice

- 2 tablespoons olive oil

- 1 small onion, finely chopped

- 2 cloves garlic, minced

- 2 cups low-sodium vegetable broth

- 1 teaspoon dried thyme

- 1 teaspoon dried rosemary

- Salt and pepper to taste

- Chopped fresh parsley for garnish (optional)

Prep Steps:

Rinse and Soak Rice:

Rinse brown rice under cold water. Soak rice in water for 15-20 minutes, then drain.

Sauté Aromatics:

In a saucepan, heat olive oil over medium heat. Sauté chopped onion until translucent, then add minced garlic and cook for an additional minute.

Add Rice and Herbs:

Add the soaked and drained brown rice to the saucepan. Stir in dried thyme and rosemary. Cook for 2-3 minutes to toast the rice.

Pour Broth:

Pour in low-sodium vegetable broth. Season with salt and pepper according to taste.

Simmer:

Bring the mixture to a boil, then reduce heat to low, cover, and simmer for 25-30 minutes or until the rice is tender and the liquid is absorbed.

Fluff and Garnish:

Once cooked, fluff the rice with a fork. Garnish with chopped fresh parsley if desired.

Nutritional Value (per serving):

- Calories: 180 kcal
- Protein: 4g
- Fat: 5g
- Carbohydrates: 32g
- Fiber: 3g
- Sodium: 150mg
- Potassium: 120mg
- Phosphorus: 80mg

Note:

Herbed Brown Rice Pilaf is a kidney-friendly side dish rich in fiber and flavor. The aromatic blend of thyme and rosemary adds depth without increasing sodium. Adjust the herbs to your taste preferences. Serve this pilaf alongside grilled vegetables or a lean protein for a well-rounded meal. As with any dietary changes, consult with a healthcare professional or dietitian to ensure it aligns with your specific renal requirements.

Egg White Omelette with Spinach and Tomatoes

Prep Time: 15 minutes

Ingredients:

- 4 large egg whites
- 1 cup fresh spinach, chopped
- 1/2 cup cherry tomatoes, halved
- 2 tablespoons onion, finely chopped
- 1 tablespoon olive oil
- Salt and pepper to taste
- Fresh herbs (such as parsley or chives) for garnish (optional)

Prep Steps:

Prepare Vegetables:

Chop spinach, tomatoes, and onion.

Sauté Vegetables:

In a non-stick skillet, heat olive oil over medium heat. Sauté chopped onion until softened. Add spinach and tomatoes, cooking until spinach wilts and tomatoes soften.

Whisk Egg Whites:

In a bowl, whisk the egg whites until slightly frothy. Season with salt and pepper.

Pour Egg Whites:

Pour the whisked egg whites over the sautéed vegetables in the skillet.

Cook Omelette:

Allow the egg whites to set at the edges. Gently lift the edges with a spatula, tilting the skillet to let the uncooked egg flow to the edges.

Add Vegetables:

Once the omelette is mostly set, add the sautéed spinach, tomatoes, and onion to one side.

Fold and Serve:

Carefully fold the omelette in half, covering the vegetables. Slide it onto a plate and garnish with fresh herbs if desired.

Nutritional Value (per serving):

- Calories: 120 kcal
- Protein: 15g
- Fat: 5g
- Carbohydrates: 5g
- Fiber: 2g
- Sodium: 180mg
- Potassium: 300mg
- Phosphorus: 120mg

Note:

This Egg White Omelette with Spinach and Tomatoes is a kidney-friendly breakfast option, low in phosphorus and rich in protein. The omission of egg yolks reduces phosphorus content. Customize with your favorite low-potassium vegetables and herbs. Pair it with whole grain toast for a balanced meal. As with any dietary changes, consult with a healthcare professional or dietitian to ensure it aligns with your specific renal requirements.

Cucumber Avocado Salad

Prep Time: 15 minutes

Ingredients:

- 2 medium cucumbers, thinly sliced
- 2 ripe avocados, diced
- 1 cup cherry tomatoes, halved
- 1/4 cup red onion, thinly sliced
- 2 tablespoons fresh cilantro, chopped
- 1 tablespoon olive oil
- 1 tablespoon lime juice
- Salt and pepper to taste
- Optional: Feta cheese for garnish

Prep Steps:

Prepare Vegetables:

Wash and slice cucumbers, dice avocados, halve cherry tomatoes, thinly slice red onion, and chop fresh cilantro.

Combine Ingredients:

In a large bowl, combine sliced cucumbers, diced avocados, halved cherry tomatoes, sliced red onion, and chopped cilantro.

Make Dressing:

In a small bowl, whisk together olive oil, lime juice, salt, and pepper to create the dressing.

Toss Salad:

Pour the dressing over the salad ingredients and gently toss to coat evenly.

Chill (Optional):

If desired, refrigerate the salad for 15-20 minutes to allow the flavors to meld.

Garnish and Serve:

Optionally, garnish with crumbled feta cheese before serving. Serve chilled.

Nutritional Value (per serving):

- Calories: 180 kcal
- Protein: 3g
- Fat: 15g
- Carbohydrates: 12g
- Fiber: 7g
- Sodium: 15mg
- Potassium: 650mg
- Phosphorus: 80mg

Note:

This Cucumber Avocado Salad is a refreshing and kidney-friendly dish. Avocado provides healthy fats, while cucumber and tomatoes add freshness. The lime dressing enhances the flavors without increasing sodium. Adjust salt according to your dietary needs. Enjoy this salad as a side or a light meal. As with any dietary changes, consult with a healthcare professional or dietitian to ensure it aligns with your specific renal requirements.

Baked Cod with Herbed Tomato Sauce

Prep Time: 25 minutes

Ingredients:

- 4 cod fillets (about 6 ounces each)
- 2 cups cherry tomatoes, halved
- 2 cloves garlic, minced
- 1 tablespoon olive oil
- 1 teaspoon dried oregano
- 1 teaspoon dried basil
- 1/2 teaspoon dried thyme
- Salt and pepper to taste
- Fresh basil leaves for garnish

Prep Steps:

Preheat Oven:

Preheat your oven to 375°F (190°C).

Prepare Cod Fillets:

Pat the cod fillets dry with a paper towel and place them in a baking dish.

Make Herbed Tomato Sauce:

In a bowl, combine halved cherry tomatoes, minced garlic, olive oil, dried oregano, dried basil, dried thyme, salt, and pepper. Toss to coat the tomatoes in the herbs.

Top Cod with Tomato Sauce:

Spoon the herbed tomato mixture over the cod fillets, ensuring they are well-covered.

Bake:

Bake in the preheated oven for 20-25 minutes or until the cod is opaque and flakes easily with a fork.

Garnish and Serve:

Remove from the oven, garnish with fresh basil leaves, and serve hot.

Nutritional Value (per serving):

- Calories: 180 kcal
- Protein: 25g
- Fat: 7g
- Carbohydrates: 5g
- Fiber: 2g
- Sodium: 150mg
- Potassium: 600mg
- Phosphorus: 220mg

Note:

Baked Cod with Herbed Tomato Sauce is a kidney-friendly and flavorful dish. The combination of herbs and tomatoes adds zest without excess sodium. Ensure the cod is sourced from reliable places to maintain freshness. Serve this dish with a side of steamed vegetables or a low-potassium grain for a balanced meal. As with any dietary changes, consult with a healthcare professional or dietitian to ensure it aligns with your specific renal requirements.

Asparagus and Almond Stir-Fry

Prep Time: 20 minutes

Ingredients:

- 1 bunch asparagus, trimmed and cut into 2-inch pieces
- 1/2 cup sliced almonds
- 2 tablespoons olive oil
- 2 cloves garlic, minced
- 1 teaspoon low-sodium soy sauce
- 1 teaspoon rice vinegar
- 1 teaspoon honey or maple syrup
- Sesame seeds for garnish (optional)
- Salt and pepper to taste

Prep Steps:

Blanch Asparagus:

Bring a pot of water to a boil. Blanch asparagus for 2-3 minutes until just tender. Drain and set aside.

Toast Almonds:

In a dry skillet, toast sliced almonds over medium heat until golden brown. Remove from the skillet and set aside.

Sauté Garlic:

In the same skillet, heat olive oil over medium heat. Sauté minced garlic until fragrant but not browned.

Stir-Fry Asparagus:

Add blanched asparagus to the skillet. Stir-fry for 2-3 minutes until coated in garlic-infused oil.

Prepare Sauce:

In a small bowl, mix low-sodium soy sauce, rice vinegar, and honey (or maple syrup).

Combine and Toss:

Pour the sauce over the asparagus. Toss to coat evenly.

Add Almonds and Garnish:

Add the toasted almonds to the stir-fry. Toss again. Garnish with sesame seeds if desired.

Nutritional Value (per serving):

- Calories: 150 kcal
- Protein: 6g

- Fat: 12g

- Carbohydrates: 8g

- Fiber: 4g

- Sodium: 90mg

- Potassium: 300mg

- Phosphorus: 90mg

Note:

Asparagus and Almond Stir-Fry is a kidney-friendly, nutrient-packed dish. Asparagus provides fiber, and almonds add a satisfying crunch. Adjust the sweetness and saltiness to suit your taste. Serve it over brown rice or quinoa for a complete meal. Always consult with a healthcare professional or dietitian to ensure it aligns with your specific renal requirements.

Low-Phosphorus Berry Smoothie

Prep Time: 10 minutes

Ingredients:

- 1/2 cup blueberries (fresh or frozen)

- 1/2 cup strawberries, hulled (fresh or frozen)

- 1/2 cup raspberries (fresh or frozen)

- 1/2 banana, sliced

- 1 cup unsweetened almond milk (or any low-phosphorus milk alternative)

- 1/2 cup ice cubes

- 1 tablespoon chia seeds (optional)

- 1 tablespoon honey or maple syrup (optional for sweetness)

Prep Steps:

Prepare Berries:

If using fresh berries, wash them thoroughly. Hull the strawberries and slice the banana.

Combine Ingredients:

In a blender, combine blueberries, strawberries, raspberries, sliced banana, almond milk, and ice cubes.

Add Chia Seeds (Optional):

For added fiber and omega-3 fatty acids, you can add chia seeds to the blender.

Blend Until Smooth:

Blend all the ingredients until you achieve a smooth and creamy consistency.

Taste and Sweeten (Optional):

Taste the smoothie and add honey or maple syrup if additional sweetness is desired. Blend again to combine.

Serve Cold:

Pour the smoothie into a glass and serve cold.

Nutritional Value (per serving):

- Calories: 150 kcal

- Protein: 3g

- Fat: 5g

- Carbohydrates: 25g

- Fiber: 7g

- Sodium: 80mg

- Potassium: 280mg

- Phosphorus: 80mg

Note:

This Low-Phosphorus Berry Smoothie is a kidney-friendly and delicious way to enjoy the goodness of berries. The recipe uses low-phosphorus fruits and almond milk. Adjust the sweetness based on your preference and dietary needs. The addition of chia seeds provides extra nutritional benefits. Consult with a healthcare professional or dietitian to ensure it aligns with your specific renal requirements.

Roasted Brussels Sprouts with Lemon Zest:

Prep Time: 30 minutes

Ingredients:

- 1 pound Brussels sprouts, trimmed and halved

- 2 tablespoons olive oil

- 1 teaspoon garlic powder

- Salt and pepper to taste

- Zest of 1 lemon

- 2 tablespoons fresh parsley, chopped (for garnish)

Prep Steps:

Preheat Oven:

Preheat your oven to 400°F (200°C).

Prepare Brussels Sprouts:

Trim the ends of the Brussels sprouts and cut them in half.

Coat with Olive Oil:

In a mixing bowl, toss the Brussels sprouts with olive oil, ensuring they are evenly coated.

Season:

Sprinkle garlic powder, salt, and pepper over the Brussels sprouts. Toss again to distribute the seasonings.

Roast in Oven:

Spread the Brussels sprouts on a baking sheet in a single layer. Roast in the preheated oven for 20-25 minutes or until they are golden brown and crisp at the edges.

Zest Lemon:

While the Brussels sprouts are roasting, zest one lemon.

Finish and Garnish:

Once the Brussels sprouts are done, transfer them to a serving dish. Sprinkle lemon zest over the top and garnish with fresh chopped parsley.

Nutritional Value (per serving):

- Calories: 120 kcal
- Protein: 4g
- Fat: 7g
- Carbohydrates: 14g
- Fiber: 7g
- Sodium: 30mg
- Potassium: 480mg
- Phosphorus: 80mg

Note:

These Roasted Brussels Sprouts with Lemon Zest are a kidney-friendly side dish with a burst of citrusy flavor. The high fiber content supports a kidney-friendly diet. Adjust the seasonings to your preference. Serve alongside a lean protein source for a balanced meal. As with any dietary changes, consult with a healthcare professional or dietitian to ensure it aligns with your specific renal requirements.

Turkey Lettuce Wraps

Prep Time: 20 minutes

Ingredients:

- 1 pound ground turkey
- 1 tablespoon olive oil
- 1 small onion, finely diced
- 2 cloves garlic, minced
- 1 teaspoon ground ginger
- 1 teaspoon low-sodium soy sauce
- 1 teaspoon rice vinegar
- 1/2 teaspoon sesame oil
- 1/2 cup water chestnuts, finely chopped
- 1/4 cup green onions, sliced
- 1 head iceberg or butter lettuce, leaves separated

Prep Steps:

Cook Ground Turkey:

In a skillet over medium heat, cook ground turkey until browned. Drain excess fat if necessary.

Sauté Aromatics:

In the same skillet, add olive oil, diced onion, minced garlic, and ground ginger. Sauté until the onion is translucent.

Season Turkey:

Add low-sodium soy sauce, rice vinegar, and sesame oil to the cooked turkey. Stir well to coat.

Add Water Chestnuts and Green Onions:

Mix in finely chopped water chestnuts and sliced green onions. Cook for an additional 2-3 minutes until heated through.

Assemble Lettuce Wraps:

Spoon the turkey mixture into individual lettuce leaves, creating wraps.

Serve:

Arrange the lettuce wraps on a serving platter and serve immediately.

Nutritional Value (per serving):

- Calories: 180 kcal
- Protein: 20g
- Fat: 8g
- Carbohydrates: 8g
- Fiber: 2g
- Sodium: 180mg
- Potassium: 300mg
- Phosphorus: 160mg

Note:

These Turkey Lettuce Wraps are a kidney-friendly alternative to traditional wraps, using lettuce leaves instead of tortillas. The ground turkey provides lean protein, and water chestnuts add crunch. Adjust the seasoning to your taste preferences. Serve these wraps as a light and nutritious meal. As with any dietary changes, consult with a healthcare professional or dietitian to ensure it aligns with your specific renal requirements.

Broccoli and Carrot Slaw

Prep Time: 15 minutes

Ingredients:

- 2 cups broccoli florets, finely chopped
- 1 cup shredded carrots
- 1/4 cup red onion, finely chopped
- 1/4 cup raisins
- 1/4 cup sunflower seeds
- 1/2 cup low-fat mayonnaise or Greek yogurt
- 1 tablespoon apple cider vinegar
- 1 tablespoon honey
- Salt and pepper to taste

Prep Steps:

Prepare Vegetables:

Finely chop broccoli florets, shred carrots, and finely chop red onion.

Combine Vegetables:

In a large bowl, combine chopped broccoli, shredded carrots, chopped red onion, raisins, and sunflower seeds.

Make Dressing:

In a small bowl, whisk together low-fat mayonnaise or Greek yogurt, apple cider vinegar, honey, salt, and pepper to create the dressing.

Toss Slaw:

Pour the dressing over the vegetables in the large bowl. Toss the slaw until all ingredients are well-coated.

Chill (Optional):

If time allows, refrigerate the slaw for 15-20 minutes to enhance the flavors.

Serve:

Serve the broccoli and carrot slaw as a refreshing side dish.

Nutritional Value (per serving):

- Calories: 120 kcal
- Protein: 3g
- Fat: 7g
- Carbohydrates: 14g
- Fiber: 3g
- Sodium: 150mg
- Potassium: 300mg
- Phosphorus: 60mg

Note:

This Broccoli and Carrot Slaw is a kidney-friendly, crunchy delight. The combination of broccoli, carrots, and sunflower seeds provides texture and nutrients. The dressing adds a touch of sweetness without excess sodium. Customize the slaw with your favorite nuts or seeds. Enjoy it as a side or as a topping for sandwiches and wraps. As with any dietary changes, consult with a healthcare professional or dietitian to ensure it aligns with your specific renal requirements.

Low-Sodium Minestrone Soup

Prep Time: 20 minutes

Ingredients:

- 1 tablespoon olive oil
- 1 cup onion, finely chopped
- 2 cloves garlic, minced
- 1 cup celery, diced
- 1 cup carrots, diced
- 1 cup zucchini, diced
- 1 cup green beans, cut into bite-sized pieces
- 1 can (14 ounces) low-sodium diced tomatoes
- 4 cups low-sodium vegetable broth
- 2 cups water
- 1/2 cup whole wheat pasta, small shapes
- 1 can (15 ounces) low-sodium kidney beans, drained and rinsed
- 1 teaspoon dried oregano
- 1 teaspoon dried basil
- Salt and pepper to taste
- 1 cup fresh spinach, chopped
- 2 tablespoons fresh parsley, chopped (for garnish)

- Grated Parmesan cheese (optional, for serving)

Prep Steps:

Sauté Aromatics:

In a large pot, heat olive oil over medium heat. Add chopped onion and minced garlic. Sauté until onions are softened.

Add Vegetables:

Add diced celery, carrots, zucchini, and green beans to the pot. Cook for 5-7 minutes until the vegetables begin to soften.

Combine Tomatoes and Broth:

Pour in the low-sodium diced tomatoes, low-sodium vegetable broth, and water. Stir well.

Add Pasta and Beans:

Stir in the whole wheat pasta and drained kidney beans. Season with dried oregano, dried basil, salt, and pepper.

Simmer:

Bring the soup to a boil, then reduce the heat to low. Cover and simmer for 10-12 minutes or until the pasta and vegetables are tender.

Add Spinach:

Stir in the chopped fresh spinach and cook until wilted.

Garnish and Serve:

Ladle the soup into bowls. Garnish with fresh parsley and, if desired, grated Parmesan cheese.

Nutritional Value (per serving):

- Calories: 180 kcal
- Protein: 8g
- Fat: 4g
- Carbohydrates: 30g
- Fiber: 8g
- Sodium: 150mg
- Potassium: 600mg
- Phosphorus: 120mg

Note:

This Low-Sodium Minestrone Soup is kidney-friendly, packed with vegetables, and low in sodium. The whole wheat pasta and kidney beans provide a good source of fiber and protein. Adjust the seasoning according to your taste preferences. Serve this soup as a hearty and nutritious meal, and feel free to customize with additional low-potassium vegetables. Always consult with a healthcare professional or dietitian to ensure it aligns with your specific renal requirements.

CONCLUSION

In this kidney-conscious cookbook, every recipe is a testament to the harmonious blend of flavor and renal wellness. Each meticulously crafted dish transforms dietary restrictions into a celebration of taste, proving that health-conscious eating need not sacrifice culinary delight. From vibrant salads to hearty mains, every recipe is a journey, not only through the diverse world of flavors but towards a nourished and thriving life.

This cookbook transcends the realm of mere recipes; it's a guide, a companion in the pursuit of well-being. It illuminates the path to renal health, making every meal a deliberate and delicious step toward a balanced life. With creativity in the kitchen, thoughtful ingredient choices, and a focus on nutritional balance, this collection not only satisfies the palate but also empowers individuals to take charge of their health. For those navigating the intricacies of renal care, this cookbook is more than a culinary compendium; it's an invitation to savor life, one kidney-friendly dish at a time.